Table of Contents

The Connection Between Autism and Irritable Bowel Syndrome: A Comprehensive Analysis

IBS and Autism: Exploring Digestive Issues in ASD

1. Introduction to Autism Spectrum Disorder (ASD) and Irritable Bowel Syndrome (IBS)

Although significant research has been conducted investigating the co-occurrence of mental health problems and ASD, no studies have yet looked in-depth at IBS or explored the relationship between ASD and IBS. Gastrointestinal problems are frequently reported by individuals with ASD with unmet needs in the treatment of digestive problems. Addressing the high rates of gastrointestinal problems experienced by individuals with ASD is an important and neglected area requiring exploration.

IBS and ASD have a range of common features. For example, both conditions are more common in women and girls than in men and boys. Studies have also suggested that people with ASD and IBS may have more severe symptoms than people without ASD, and that some of the ways in which they think and feel about their symptoms are not the same as those without ASD.

Irritable bowel syndrome (IBS) is a common, but poorly understood, condition. IBS affects the large bowel (colon) and leads to symptoms like abdominal pain, bloating, constipation, and diarrhea. It can occur at any age, but commonly first starts during the teenage years and twenties.

Autism Spectrum Disorder (ASD) is a lifelong neurodevelopmental condition. People with ASD have difficulties with social communication and social interaction, and typically experience restricted, repetitive patterns of behavior. Approximately three-quarters of people with ASD have a co-occurring condition, also known as a 'comorbidity'. This includes medical conditions like allergies, asthma, and irritable bowel syndrome.

2. Prevalence and Co-occurrence of IBS in Individuals with ASD

The gastrointestinal tract and its function have received increasing attention in ASD. The points at issue range from the description on particular complaints such as functional constipation to conceptual ideas such as the gut-brain axis and even touch the level of proposed pathophysiology. In the meantime, this organelle has become interesting as a therapeutic target, as indicated by some controlled treatment outcome trials and also in the ASD field. The prevalence of IBS has been reported to be higher in ASD populations than in the general population. The prevalence of IBS in ASD is reported to be between 8.0% and 9.6% in Korean ASD cohorts. This is in line with the prevalence of 9.6% in the general population and the prevalence among Danish pediatric ASD patients of 10.8%. In the Korean general populations, 70% of the IBS cases were women, while in the ASD population, the majority, 57.1%, was male. In an Italian study, high-functioning adult patients had a prevalence of IBS of 18.7% and a further 20% fulfilled the Rome III criteria for subthreshold IBS, that is IBS in remission.

The comorbid occurrence of pervasive developmental disorders (PDD) or Autism Spectrum Disorder (ASD) with gastrointestinal symptoms has been increasingly reported in the past decade. The highest frequency has been reported in the area of functional disorders of gut-brain interaction (DGBI) such as functional constipation and irritable bowel syndrome (IBS). In a study from Denmark, Christiansen and co-workers reported that Danish pediatric patients with ASD were six times more likely to have IBS and/or functional constipation than the general population. The reported prevalence of IBS in the ASD population is between 1% and 50%. There are small studies of adults with ASD that have found a differential distribution of diagnostic subtypes of IBS in the ASD inpatients, with significantly less mixed IBS and IBS-constipation but significantly more IBS-diarrhea. In spite of substantial methodological problems, the current data indicate that IBS is not only over-represented in the entire field of DGBI but also in the ASD population which also bases on biological and clinical grounds.

3. Common Gastrointestinal Symptoms in ASD

Whether individuals with ASD are more prone to develop the symptoms of IBD remains an open question, especially as typical presentations of IBD include anemia that's underdiagnosed in individuals with extensive disability, arthritis with gait alterations that could be ignored in people with neurological disorders such as cerebral palsy and ASD, and rectal bleeding that might not be communicable in people with problems of expressive language. In sum, individuals with ASD and gastrointestinal complaints seem to have gastrointestinal symptoms, but not other problems or immunological issues that seem to be objectively measured as more prevalent in generalized widespread pain and IBD. It would be essential to follow children from performance-based with and without gastrointestinal complaints to investigate to what extent gastrointestinal problems would interfere with cognition, language, and performance on the whole.

Since the gastrointestinal manifestations in people with ASD seem to be heterogeneous with various biological, anatomical, immunological, neurological, and physiological underpinnings, it is odd that physical or neurological findings are ignored in favor of a diagnosis of IBS/IBD upon a pain description. A quarter to more than a half of individuals with ASD and GI complaints would be diagnosed with IBS compared to the general population. The risk of having IBD was much less than in the control population, and was the same as in people not presenting with abdominal pain in a study of more than 600 young adults; most people presenting with IBD or IBS indicated no abdominal pain.

Gastrointestinal Symptoms in ASD Independent of a Diagnosed Disorder Several studies suggest that gastrointestinal disorders could be a more frequent comorbidity in patients with ASD. A significant number of patients were reported to suffer from abdominal pain, gastrointestinal infections, and food and other allergies; the most commonly suspected allergen was gluten, a tissue with alleged immunogenic and opiate-like properties. It was concluded that dietary modifications and increased iron intake did not have any general long-term effects on the behavior or cognitive functions of the patients.

In at least 20% of children and adults with ASD, more than one coexisting condition can be identified. Regrettably, gastrointestinal symptoms in individuals with ASD can go clinically unnoticed or remain unexplored because an element of the broader phenotype is to be non-specific and have more variable presentations than in the typically developing population. Troubleshooting GI symptoms in individuals with ASD can be challenging because of comorbid issues such as sensory and motor impairments, comorbid medical and metabolic issues such as epilepsy and immune disorders, the use of atypical medication, and the inability of the person with ASD to provide accurate self-reports.

Gastrointestinal (GI) symptoms are one of the most commonly reported comorbidities in Autism Spectrum Disorder (ASD) and can manifest as abdominal pain (up to 49% of individuals with ASD) and discomfort, bloating, diarrhea, constipation (which seems to be especially common), gastroesophageal reflux, vomiting, or fecal incontinence. In addition to their significant negative impact on the quality of life of the individual with ASD, these symptoms can also contribute to an exacerbation of problem behavior.

4. Potential Causes and Mechanisms of Digestive Issues in ASD

What are the potential mechanisms contributing to the pain pathway in ASD? ASD requires further exploration to confirm hypotheses about connections between co-occurring complaints and the peculiarities of genetic code, including differential expression (DE) of particular genes. It is necessary to mention that IBS and digestive issues in ASD are multifactorial and result from a complex interplay among genetics, environmental factors (e.g., diet and infections), the gastrointestinal (GI) microbiota, and other co-occurring health complaints. These imply dietary nutrients that may have a poor cross into the CNS, hormones stimulating the CNS to regulate mood, and the hormones' actual transformation. It is interesting to note that, in general, psychological stress or GI discomfort set off a cyclic process. For example, anxiety and depression can lead to GI symptoms, which cause pain followed by sleep loss and emotional disturbances. The opposite is also observed as GI infections or chronic pain causes mood tied to IBS. Although the existence of more cycles is suggested above, a person will often seek medical attention for the initial pain and complaint. In our discussion here, we present a model that explains one of the altered CNS pathways. Always keep in mind that it is a hypothesis of the findings presented.

What are the potential triggers for digestive issues in ASD? There have been many explanations as to why approximately 10.5-80% of people diagnosed with ASD experience digestive issues. One hypothesis is that both populations may have more sensitive digestive systems. Another popular hypothesis is that many people with ASD have gluten sensitivity or an allergy to casein that is sometimes a part of celiac disease. These are thought to be correlates rather than main contributors to GI issues. However, many studies have shown scientifically that a gluten-free (GF) diet can help with some of the symptoms seen in ASD such as trouble sleeping and hyperactive behavior. Thus, a lack of scientifically based relationships between particular physiological states may not preclude the treatment of those symptoms seen in ASD. The biome has also been well studied in connection with the functioning of one of the enteric nervous systems (ENS) and the central nervous system (CNS) as well as developing behaviors usually associated with the disease state.

4. Potential Causes and Mechanisms of Digestive Issues in ASD.

Digestive issues. Pitfalls in the prepping caregiver. IBS and Autism: Exploring Digestive Issues in ASD.

5. Impact of Digestive Issues on Individuals with ASD

Gastrointestinal (GI) disturbances have been reported as common in the autism population, with typically co-occurring issues such as sleep disturbances, cognitive impairments and challenging behavior. In typical populations, chronic illness in general is negatively associated with quality of life indicative of a high priority for those in the autism population with GI complaints. Quantification of the psychophysiological distress imposed by such complaints, as measured via physiological and behavioral reactivity (e.g., increased pain responsiveness, sleep disturbances) may further suggest the negative impact of these associated problems on individuals' overall functioning.

The combination of an autism spectrum disorder and enuresis may interfere with the skills necessary to be successful in the kindergarten years of children. Children need to be free of diapers before they enroll in kindergarten school. Additionally, the odor of urine and feces may interfere with typical social experiences and increase bullying by other children in schools. Children with an autism spectrum disorder may be at greater risk than children without a disability of physical, emotional or sexual abuse. Additionally, approximately 30 percent of children with any disabilities (including autism) are reportedly abused in some way.

In a previous study, parents of 152 Israeli children with ASD reported significantly more behavioral disorders such as aggression, irritability, anxiety, stereotypy, and hyperactivity after suffering a bout of diarrhea than did parents of 159 children with a developmental disability. Delays in independent toileting skills (elimination) were reported up to four times more often for children with an autism spectrum disorder than children without.

As per Mahapatra and Chittleborough, children with an autism spectrum disorder tend to have significant difficulty with removing waste from their body including both urinating and bowel movements. Up to 83 percent of children with an ASD have enuresis or nocturnal enuresis or encopresis.

In a study that assessed the communication and social skills among 878 children with Autism Spectrum Disorder (ASD), 70 percent of children with ASD reportedly had issues with digestion. Earlier evidence has been supportive of the fact that individuals with ASD tend to experience a higher rate of certain physical (e.g., peptic ulcer disease, gastritis, lactose intolerance, and chronic diarrhea) and emotional problems, including fear, anxiety, extreme anger, panic, and stress. Additionally, people with Asperger syndrome, one of the conditions under ASD in the DSM-5, are noted to experience more gastrointestinal problems compared to controls.

6. Assessment and Diagnosis of Digestive Issues in Individuals with ASD

The process of recognizing symptoms and understanding the problem areas is challenging. All of us have our own digestive issues, but we often do not pay much attention to details or pay close attention to little things that happen to us every day (i.e., being bloated, having gas, eating the wrong thing at times). The difficult thing is to separate the truly significant symptoms from common, rarely problematic conditions. Lastly, it also is important to recognize that for any assessment of possible digestive problems in an individual with ASD an "individualized" approach is taken into consideration, recognizing that one style of concern might not pertain to others. Each area tends to have its own concerns and compact quite differently. Everyone carries their own label. There are two key points about this process: it is very individualized, and it is very complex. The best approach is to see initial medical evaluation with a specialist that is familiar with both ASD and co-occurring digestive issues. That, however, is not always possible, and this field is complex and new. It can also be reasonable to seek a developmental specialist familiar with ASD and engage in a basic evaluation to set up the stage for more careful evaluation. Make time and be prepared for a long assessment with continual follow-up care.

Because of many complex issues surrounding the digestive tracts of many individuals with Autism Spectrum Disorder

(ASD), we are quite serious about exploring problems that can occur in these areas in our web project. It is our hope that, with additional research and understanding, new treatment options can be developed. This section is devoted to explaining the assessment and diagnosis of these various problems that tend to occur in individuals with Autism Spectrum Disorder. The process used for this clinical evaluation is that professionals must work carefully through a variety of possibilities and then realize that the diagnostic process is never really complete. It takes a very long, careful, and detailed evaluation to see if any symptoms present are significant enough for a diagnosis. This careful examination is certainly more complex— children with ASD are more likely to fall through diagnostic cracks. It is our hope that funding for additional research in this critical area of assessment brings some clarity and understanding to effective assessment tools.

7. Management and Treatment Strategies for IBS in Individuals with ASD

As previously mentioned, IBS is a medical disorder. Therefore, treatment from medical health professionals may be warranted. Many medical professionals are aware of the predisposition between autism and IBS; however, they may not be equipped to address some of the behaviors that come with IBS (i.e., attempting to defecate on the floor in the classroom, muscular relaxation when pressed to defecate). Moreover, most gastroenterologists are unable to fully address the behaviors related to IBS that children with autism have. Thus, the treatment of IBS in a child with autism may need to be a multidisciplinary approach, including physician services (i.e., gastroenterologist, speech and language therapist, and physical and emotional therapist). This requires a team that can include a neuropediatrician, nutritional doctor, occupational therapist, a psychiatrist or psychologist, and a speech therapist in addition to polyspecialized pediatricians. Treatment for a subset of children with autism might consist of educating the patients. Treatment strategies include dietary intervention, medication, special equipment, operant conditioning, operant biofeedback, and rotation diets. Treatment plans must be individualized and adapted to each patient's symptoms and learning abilities. A good treatment plan must take into account the basis of the child's autism while centering on the gastrointestinal tract. Effective home and group management strategies include daily routines, a safe quiet place, diet to lessen factors that irritate the bowel, clean them, uncomfortable movements in attention span and behavior be answered with positive reinforcement, decrease stress by educating students about their disorder and about their program, the use of visual supports, creating a social story or a mini-project for the child who is able to do some self-exploration, and the child and the teachers being sensitive to bowel movements, the child's position while sitting down, and the child's motor behaviors.

Individuals with Autism Spectrum Disorder (ASD) are also known to have a higher prevalence of gastroenterological complaints, such as constipation, diarrhea, acid reflux, gastro-oesophageal reflux disease (GORD), pain, and irritable bowel syndrome (IBS). This section explores various strategies to manage and address IBS in individuals with ASD.

8. Dietary Interventions and Nutritional Considerations for Individuals with ASD and IBS

Unfortunately, evidence-based dietary interventions for individuals with co-occurring IBS or in the general ASD population need further study to make any definitive recommendations. At this time, evidence and expert opinion suggest individualizing nutritional support and providing comprehensive nutritional education and resources to adults and families. Since people with co-occurring ASD and IBS are more likely to experience several digestive issues, further studies of dietary interventions in the IBS population may be relevant and potentially impactful for this clinical group. Furthermore, they may provide system-wide and psychological benefits to certain sub-populations of individuals with Autism Spectrum Disorder.

Preliminary evidence suggests that the Specific Carbohydrate Diet (SCD), low Fermentable, Oligosaccharides, Disaccharides, Monosaccharides and Polyols (FODMAP) diet, low oxalate diet, gluten-free and/or casein-free diet (GFCF), ketogenic diet, low dose naltrexone or Buvaisar protocol may be helpful for some individuals with ASD. Nutrient requirements and specific nutritional abnormalities have been reported in the population with ASD. Several nutrient-related genetic polymorphisms have been identified in the ASD population. Digestive issues are common in ASD with prevalence estimates as high as 70%. Some digestive issues within the ASD population are known to be associated with dietary triggers. The prevalence of Irritable Bowel Syndrome (IBS) in the ASD population is estimated at over 15%. Gut microbiome disturbances are thought to potentially be associated with the pathophysiology of both ASD and IBS. IBS is a diagnosis of exclusion based on the Rome IV criteria.

Dietary interventions and nutritional considerations for individuals with Autism Spectrum Disorder (ASD) and co-occurring Irritable Bowel Syndrome (IBS)

9. Psychological and Behavioral Interventions for Managing Digestive Issues in ASD

Evidence suggests that these practices may be specifically tailored for individuals with ASD, but the study did not explore the application of stress management techniques among a subset of individuals with gastrointestinal distress. Other interventions for individuals without ASD who exhibit physiological conditions in response to anxiety, or IBS, or other irritable bowel syndromes that have evidence for efficacy among the general population include cognitive-behavioral therapy, relaxation, hypnotherapy, complementary therapies, psychodynamically based treatments, or interpersonal therapy for IBS relief or stress management. These treatments target attributional styles, cognitive distortions, selective attention to bowel sensations, and the ability to ignore other interoceptive sensations while centralizing the distress or to modify physiological responses. Since the techniques are applicable outside the ASD population, stress management for adults with ASD who experience IBS may show some degree of effective modification in reducing physiological arousal that contributes to distress if the same IBS measurements are present and intellectual disability is not. Often efficacy rates are lower when applied to a general subclinical population.

Biological approaches to treating individuals with autism spectrum disorder (ASD) who experience digestive issues span dietary modification to pharmacological medications. While constipation may be a concern for individuals with idiopathic inflammatory bowel disease (IBS) and ASD, other interventions beyond biological approaches are necessary to address additional concerns related to stress, anxiety, and socio-communicative disturbances. We present current knowledge behind psychological and behavioral interventions targeting these issues in ASD. Forks given with a meal that are designed to carry a visual image of digestion with a brief verbal explanation about the food that will be coming serve to face the maladaptive preferences of photos of the Meals on the Fork Show the Reasons (MoFSR) in autism spectrum disorder (ASD) and are effective in increasing food consumption in the ASD population.

27. Psychological and behavioral interventions, including cognitive-behavioral therapy for digestive issues in autism spectrum disorder

10. Current Research and Future Directions in Understanding the Relationship between ASD and IBS

It is suggested that there are four key areas of research that are likely to herald advancements in our understanding of the relationship between ASD and IBS in the short term. These areas include re-conceptualizing gastrointestinal (GI) presentation in ASD, the role of the microbiome, the use of suitable tools for measuring the underlying phenotype of stress and generalized anxiety, and a more thorough biological understanding of the biological, particularly neurological, alterations that manifest in both conditions. There is consensus about autism being on a spectrum or continuum. It is proposed that domain-wide weakness, including a weaker non-linear trajectory in cortical neural function, underpins a spectrum of central integrative disorders from associative to lower functioning pervasive developmental disorders (PDDs) to autism. The precise shape of this trajectory is not yet resolved but thought to be non-linear in nature. Processing of afferent information within the interoceptive nervous system, convergence zone, and related nervous systems may be affected in ASD. Current knowledge of afferent and efferent processing of information within interoceptive pathways in ASD is reviewed in light of this research. Ongoing research in interoceptive information processing and transfer, analytically synthesizing ASD sensory information globally, is required. Sustainable multidisciplinary interventional models that focus on the meta-modeling of knowledge in autism are needed to improve clinical and demographic ASD outcomes. Additionally, the future must take the new phenomenology (personal language) seriously, which is known to be detailed, consistent, and profound in ASD. Evidence will be provided to justify the case. A new multidisciplinary research paradigm, "Autism as a Disorder of Interoception," will be advanced.

Over the past 150 years, the relationship between autism spectrum disorder (ASD) and non-organic bowel disturbances has been much debated. Currently, some practitioners consider that difficulties in the micro and macro environment of the bowel initiate, exacerbate, or sustain autistic characteristics. On the other hand, other researchers consider that the opposite cannot be excluded. They suggest that the high prevalence of irritable bowel syndrome (IBS), which is part of the recently conceptualized "Functional Bowel Disorders" in ASD, might be seen as a product of autism rather than a cause. However, upon closer inspection of the bulk of research to date, the ASD-IBS comorbidity is inconclusive despite the high prevalence of bowel disturbances in this population. The suggested reasons for such variability in the ASD-IBS comorbidity include informant bias in the validated diagnostic tools used, as well as publication bias. Therefore, it is suggested to revisit and re-conceptualize the relationship between ASD and both organic diseases (like coeliac disease) and non-organic Functional GI conditions.

3. Current Research and Future Directions

The Connection Between Autism and Irritable Bowel Syndrome: A Comprehensive Analysis

1. Introduction

Introduction: The objective of this article is to lay the foundation for a comprehensive neurogastroenterology investigation of the relationship between alterations in gut functioning and the development of symptoms of autism. We first review the evidence from the rapidly growing field of study of the gut-brain axis. We then review the present state of the literature on comorbidity of autism and irritable bowel syndrome (IBS). After making the case for a bidirectional relationship between autism and alterations in gut functioning and secretions, we conclude with an examination of gene expression and proteomic data. This investigation supports our hypothesis that through the effect of Oxytocin as a neuromodulator on nonlinear gut functioning, promising therapeutic approaches already being studied to improve IBS may also have a positive impact on symptoms of autism in those patients.

This article presents an extensive analysis that seeks to improve the understanding and treatment of Autism Spectrum Disorder (ASD) from the perspective of Irritable Bowel Syndrome (IBS). The ultimate objective is to test promising therapeutic approaches to improve IBS and, thereby, autism symptoms. Below, we report our review of the literature, including the existing evidence that supports a bidirectional relationship between functioning in the brain and the gut. This section is followed by the close analysis of the studies linking autism and IBS. We finally support our hypotheses with our review of the connection between the two diseases.

1.1. Background and Significance

Given the high rates of IBS and more widely defined functional abdominal pain (FAP) in children with autism, as well as the importance of examining GI symptoms in autism treatment multi-disciplinary programs, we have taken an initial cross-sectional approach to examining the relationship between autism and IBS. For a recent survey study, we investigated the extent to which irritable bowel syndrome and sub-threshold IBS occur in autism disorders. We also studied the clinical course of irritable bowel syndrome and sub-threshold IBS in autism. We used solicitation through electronic mailing lists for formal and informal practices and published lists of conferences and meetings for this study. Our detailed analysis program accounts for important age differences and describes the psychiatric features and risk for suicide associated with irritability trigger-rates in autism disorders and sub-threshold IBS.

Autism is a developmental disorder which is characterized clinically by social impairments along with repetitive patterns of behavior and the presence of narrow interests. While autism's exact etiology still remains unclear, both genetic as well as environmental factors are thought to play roles in the developmental course of the condition. A recent study in a commercially-insured pediatric population has quantified large increases in the prevalence rates of autism from less than 3.5/10,000 in the early 2000s to over 53/10,000 in 2010. Recent estimates place the overall prevalence of autism at 1.5% of the total

American population. Some of these children also experience irritable bowel syndrome (IBS). Patients with irritable bowel syndrome and autism are likely to have more severe symptoms compared to those without autism and tend to miss work more often. In autism, the severity of gastrointestinal symptoms correlate with the presence and severity of irritability. Further preliminary data indicates early life GI symptoms might distinguish two clinical subtypes of autism.

1.2. Purpose of the Study

In the present broadly reviewed systemic study, we not only aim to reveal empirical or PubMed articles demonstrating the coexistence of symptoms such as constipation, diarrhea, behavioral deficit, etc. of autism and IBS patients but also provide a comprehensive analysis of the link and putative mutual brain-gut-immune dysregulation mechanism. Additionally, the paper provides the link between autism and IBS with comorbid conditions, potential inhibition/deficit in the animal disease model of pain and anxiety, and a mechanism responsible for the negative association of behavioral deficit such as IBS with autism. Finally, genetic or environmental risk factors that could result in autism, but not with IBS, are also discussed.

Autism is a behavioral pattern genetic disorder/disability that occurs in early childhood and affects 1 out of 59 individuals born globally. As per the estimates, more than 11 million people today live with autism in India. Autism occurs due to both genetic and environmental risk factors that result in altered early brain development and lead to difficulties in social skills, repetitive behaviors, speech, and nonverbal communication. There is no exact cause of autism, and Asperger syndrome, childhood disintegrative disorder, Rett Syndrome, and pervasive developmental disorder (PDD) are a few of the conditions of autistic spectrum disorder. This disorder is not only a single symptom disorder; it is associated with many co-occurring disorders. The co-occurring disorders include neurological, psychological, and somatic disorders such as gastrointestinal disorders, IBS, food allergy, anxiety, and depression.

The present comprehensive analysis is aimed at examining the extent to which autism and IBS are connected to each other to report comparable symptoms and the putative underlying mutual brain-endocrine-immune dysregulation. It also provides potential behavioral alterations, molecule signaling proteins, pathology, medication response, and nutrition, etc.

2. Understanding Autism Spectrum Disorder (ASD)

The U.S. Centers for Disease Control and Prevention (CDC) estimate the prevalence of ASD to be 1 in 54 children in the United States, though studies have reported higher rates. Males are four times more likely than females to be diagnosed with ASD. It is unclear whether this is due to gender bias or an increased incidence of ASD in males. Although ASD is often diagnosed in childhood, it is a lifelong condition, and the needs and challenges of individuals with ASD can change over time, particularly with effective services and supports. Given the wide range of potential symptoms that can accompany ASD, no two individuals are alike. The phrase, "If you've met one person with autism, you've met one person with autism," underscores this concept. While there is no definitive list of ASD features, characteristics may include excessive fears and phobias, difficulties understanding jokes and idioms, hypersensitivity to light or touch, and a strong preference for routine and repetitive play. In some cases, an individual's mood can change without any recognizable reason, and an individual may engage in repetitive body movements, also known as "stimming."

Autism Spectrum Disorder (ASD) is a complex neurodevelopmental disorder that describes a wide range of neurobehavioral and developmental conditions. Aptly called a "spectrum," the symptoms and characteristics of ASD can present themselves in a variety of combinations and range from mild to severe. According to the Diagnostic and Statistical Manual of Mental Disorders, Fifth Edition (DSM-5), an individual need not have cognitive disability to be diagnosed with ASD. However, because individuals may demonstrate delays in, impairments of, or difficulties with social communication and interaction—which is the first main component of ASD—problems in the other two main symptom areas of restricted, repetitive patterns of behavior, interests or activities and sensory processing are also considered. Researchers within the ASD community often conceptualize these main domains of impairment as "social-communicative" and "non-social."

2.1. Definition and Diagnostic Criteria

There is presently no productive biological or genetic target to validate the presence or severity of ASD. The judgment of ASD and its severity relies on a huge amount of original or restructured clinical data, often rigid criteria. The multidisciplinary assessment typically requires a physician familiar with the characteristics of ASD, and may include developmental or pediatric neurologists or pediatricians, child or adult psychiatrists, speech pathologists, neuropsychologists, special educators, and occupational and physical therapists, etc. The identification process of the ASD varies in path-integrated hospital systems with trained units who are verifiable also in other clinical categories. The analysis appears to be different between two regions and requires well-founded and up-to-date diagnostic criteria.

Diagnostic Criteria

ASD is characterized not by a set of uniform symptoms but rather by a broad range of impairments. Nonetheless, several critical aspects unite these various expressions, including qualitative social and interpersonal weaknesses, communication and language disorders, and odd and repetitive behavior patterns. An important feature is that individuals with classic autism (Kanner) appear to be mentally retarded, whereas those with Asperger's syndrome have normal intelligence and sometimes very strong areas of strength. In order to refer to the entire spectrum, the necessary shifts have been made in the classification criteria. The term "spectrum" highlights the considerable variation in the appearance of the disturbances, grouped as typically classified in distinct types in the descriptions. In addition, it underscores some related characteristics of individuals with autistic disorder or with PDD-NOS, such as HFA and Asperger's syndrome.

Autism Spectrum Disorder

2.2. Prevalence and Characteristics

The age of first diagnosis in the global population has generally decreased from approximately 3 to 5 years in the 1980s to less than 4 years 10 years later. In Italy, data collected over 9 years have shown a latent period before diagnosis, with the earlier diagnosis in Varese (approximately between 2 and 3), which may be explained by the higher levels in social capital and social networks among care providers and family members in Varese and Modena. In any event, the age of diagnosis and treatment remains late, thus increasing the overall lifetime costs. ASD is characterized by a high degree of phenotypic heterogeneity, in parallel with a growing amount of knowledge related to the involvement of multiple impinging risk factors known to variably influence genetic and non-genetic background. In this regard, it is not surprising that 30-40% of children and adults with ASD are diagnosed with comorbid medical conditions, such as gastrointestinal diseases; these appear to be more common in ASD compared to the general population of children, affecting about 24% of the global population.

ASD is characterized by core symptoms, which may manifest with variable clinical presentations, ranging from mild to severe, as the result of executive dysfunctions related to social adaptation, communication, interests, and behavioral flexibility. Prevalence estimates have increased since the early 2000s, and according to recent data, are estimated at 1.8% of all school-age children (7 to 12 years old), with the current estimate of population prevalence compatible with the previous estimate. Among children and adolescents, a ratio is seen as about 5 boys to 1 girl.

3. Understanding Irritable Bowel Syndrome (IBS)

The methodology of measuring the prevalence of IBS in the general population is a method through which duplicate activation rates can be evaluated. When an IBS diagnosis is being performed for adult subjects under the duplicate activation technique, the disorder is reached by the exclusion from the activation technique. Any undiagnosed adults are assessed by healthcare professionals who have authored the indexing burden for gastrointestinal symptoms (IBS-IMPACT questionnaire) in Norfolk, containing 19 GI symptoms.

To unravel the prevalence and impact of IBS burden in the worldwide community, several population-based epidemiological studies have developed different techniques for defining it. It is well known that the majority of subjects with IBS seen in therapeutics also suffer from abdominal plus extra-abdominal comorbid symptoms of a different nature, with anywhere from 60%–100% reporting upper abdominal discomfort and 50%–90% reporting extra-upper GI symptoms as well. The prevalence of extra-GI symptoms is shown to be substantially higher in secondary referral IBS centers, even when compared to other FGIDs diagnosis of secondary care mixed primary and secondary care overall.

Irritable Bowel Syndrome (IBS) can be defined as chronic gastrointestinal symptom patterns which have a pervasive relation to at least one of the Criterion A symptoms: either pain related to defecation, bowel movement, or change in stool frequency or form. In clinical practice, it should be regarded as a diagnosis of inclusion. Specifically, the diagnosis of IBS should be invoked for compatibility when Criterion A is met and a full GI evaluation does not show a distinctive scientific impression. However, IBS's characteristic symptoms may be complicated by other chronic gastrointestinal disorders, particularly functional gastrointestinal diseases.

Introducing Irritable Bowel Syndrome, which is characterized by different factors. Describing the Diagnostic Criteria for Irritable Bowel Syndrome in clinical practice. Analyzing the efficient approaches to measuring the prevalence of IBS in the general population. Unraveling a comprehensive list of IBS symptoms. Introducing the Three Major classifications of IBS with the specific symptom clusters for each version of the disorder.

3. Understanding Irritable Bowel Syndrome (IBS)

3.1. Definition and Diagnostic Criteria

This questionnaire evaluates abdominal symptoms, flatus and borborygmi, and stool frequency and form in a 30-day period. In particular, IBS is preliminarily diagnosed when abdominal pain is reported at least 4 days a month. Syndrome-type IBS is further differentiated based on stool form and frequency.

The Rome Foundation suggests using these questionnaires during an initial assessment, in addition to taking a thorough medical history and performing a physical examination, to confirm or exclude a diagnosis of IBS. Patients who test positive and have no concerning symptoms should be managed conservatively, with lifestyle modifications and dietary changes. If symptoms do not improve or worsen, a patient's diagnostic evaluation may need to be broadened to exclude or confirm the presence of concomitant diseases.

Different classifications and diagnostic criteria have been proposed over the years by various organizations and experts. In particular, the Rome criteria have been updated and revised by expert consensus every decade, with the most recent revision (Rome IV) published in 2016. These criteria, defined by the Rome Foundation, can be adopted as a patient questionnaire to evaluate gastrointestinal symptoms indicative of functional bowel disorders.

Irritable bowel syndrome (IBS) is a condition characterized by abdominal pain associated with an alteration in bowel habits due to a variable combination of diarrhea and/or constipation. Patients suffering from IBS experience numerous symptoms, including excessive gas production, bloating, heartburn, dyspepsia, attention deficit, palpitations, nausea/vomiting, and muscle pain. They may also show overlap syndromes with gastroesophageal reflux, dyspepsia, anxiety, fibromyalgia, headache, and low back pain, among others.

2.2. Physiopathological Hypothesis of IBS and Its Diagnosis

2.2.1. Physiopathological Hypotheses. According to current reflections on functional gastrointestinal disorders, IBS included, proposed initially by Mayer as a biopsychosocial paradigm. The interaction between genetic, physiological, and environmental (or psychological) variables leads to the appearance of a state of dysregulation of the brain-gut axis whose characteristics are influenced by the relative weight of each of these factors.

Abdominal pain is directly correlated with colonic hyperalgesia, which is why patients with constipation have a higher expression of this symptom than those of diarrhea. Moreover, apart from the common symptoms, children present recurrences with growth alterations, loss of appetite, vomiting, tendon/muscle contractures, and low muscle tone according to patients.

Symptoms. Irritable bowel syndrome is characterized by numerous clinical alterations, from recurrent abdominal pain associated with defecation and accompanied by an alteration in bowel habit (diarrhea and/or constipation), abdominal distention, to symptoms such as incontinence of feces and flatulence. The clinical manifestations are different between males and females, with the latter showing a greater pain threshold.

Prevalence. Data obtained from good-quality studies suggest that IBS is present in 5-10% of the adult population. According to the statistical study, the prevalence of people with IBS is 2 males and 11 females per 30 people, suggesting that females are more prone to suffer from the syndrome.

4. The Overlapping Symptoms and Shared Pathophysiology

However, overlap of symptoms does not necessarily mean that both diseases have the same symptoms. In both diseases, some typical but different key symptoms are to be found, finally characterizing the primary but at the same time partly overlapping and different disturbed physiological processes that are also underlying shared and distinct symptoms. From the existing literature review and concepts, we conclude that variables linking ASD and IBS could be brain inflammation, CNS inflammation, some deregulated signal function via the endocrine system, psychiatric comorbidities, and maladaptive coping strategies.

Chronic low-grade inflammation, psychiatric comorbidities, and different subtypes of gastrointestinal diseases can be found in both ASD and IBS pathology. Moreover, rejection sensitivity, involuntary/intrusive trauma processing, or invalid negative self-statements are key symptoms which could appear typical in either of the diseases and can be a psychological problem in both. Chronic visceral or CNS inflammation could change typical brain-physiologic functions (emotional and autonomic nervous system, memory or sensory abilities) ultimately leading to some common symptoms of ASD and IBS. Maybe exactly these overlapping symptoms are also present in the few ASD patients who suffer from more severe comorbid IBS, alleviating their social functioning to a severe extent.

Irritable bowel syndrome (IBS) and autism spectrum disorder (ASD) are complex and diverse, but some common features as well as overlapped cardinal symptoms have been attributed to their pathophysiological background. The co-occurrence is also higher than the coincidental appearance found in the general population. Identification of overlapping features might possibly indicate some shared behavior in probable pathomechanisms, allowing further research essential for choosing potential novel treatment option common to both diseases. Chronic abdominal complaints have been related to brain-related symptoms and the severity of gastrointestinal symptoms correlates with the severity of autistic features.

4.1. Common Symptoms in ASD and IBS

Pathophysiology studies on both ASD and IBS have been showing a high degree of similarity in clinical presentation, as well as in respect of some biological features regarding both the central nervous system and the enteric nervous system. An Italian group recently pointed out that autistic individuals diagnosed with IBS showed a higher frequency of several GI symptoms compared to a control group with IBS only. As reported by a systematic review, subjects suffering from ASD and IBS showed significantly higher scores for general and somatic health than those with ASD only, as well as a higher daily stool frequency and score for stool consistency. On the other hand, and as expected in other series in which samples consist of adolescent to adult patients, but not in pediatric ones, a higher percentage of females with ASD and IBS presented with abdominal pain, with a possible higher expression of pain when compared with males. Besides the common pattern of expression in both autism and IBS, additional symptoms beyond the GI tract possibly depict a subgroup of subjects with both conditions. The Italian sample only showed a higher expression of non-GI symptoms such as the presence of phobias, lack of obsessions or compulsions, and sympatico-vagal imbalance. All these reported phenomenological expressions reflected increased susceptibility in ASD/IBS individuals, shared by both conditions. This is in agreement with the "intolerance to uncertainty" theory. Another plausible explanation that may justify these clinical findings might be related to the presence of multiple signaling molecules that act upon both systems and which show high expression in IBS, such as the SCF/c-KIT signaling system. In conclusion, findings from the latest epidemiologic studies, together with clinical descriptions and multi-omics tools have recently been confirming this bidirectional interaction between the brain and the gut. Rashed and co-workers, for example, already proposed an algorithm to show the association between the two conditions. In the big picture, the confusion originally observed by the fathers leading the field of classifying autism within a set of psychiatric disorders, or the latest, considering autism within the spectrum of neurodevelopmental disorders is justified.

Common symptoms in ASD and IBS. Since Kanner's first description, the so-called prototypical triad of Autism Spectrum Disorder (ASD) included several gastrointestinal symptoms, such as constipation, abdominal pain, and diarrhea, which were associated with emotional dysregulation and agitation. Health concerns related to the latter symptoms led scientists to identifying and proving an organic and non-psychological substrate for gastrointestinal (GI) symptoms in ASD. The recognition of this tract led to the identification of a clinical phenotype characterized by ASD and IBS, which is referred to as ASD/IBS.

Alteration in Gut-Brain Axis

4.2. Potential Biological Mechanisms

An expanding interest in understanding the mechanisms (genetic and environmental) of IBS and ASD at a biological basis is being characterized as the central regulator of inflammation, whose signaling affects the bidirectional feedback from brain and gut to genetic predisposition and environment to trauma experienced early on in life, also known as micro-inflammation or parental stress. Abdominal pain is well-associated with altered intestinal permeability, gut microbiome, inflammagenic signals (cytokines), brain processing networks of somatic signals as seen in IBS and non-IBS abdominal pain. The gut region is richly innervated and communicates a greater density of afferent signals to the rest of the body, including organs associated with visceral and interoception, due to the multi-meissner's and remak-sensitive density C-fibers emitting a variety of gastrointestinal-related neurotransmitters within the brain-gut/enteric nervous system (ENS).

Lack of consistent and comprehensive etiology does not invalidate the presence of shared pathophysiology between ASD and IBS. However, a probable explanation into why this shared pathophysiology has been largely unknown is that each disorder has been thought of as singular in its function and has different underlying biological processes. Overlooked is the quickly-growing field of the gut-brain axis, whose research is devoted to understanding the integrated role of the CNS and visceral inner workings in terms of endocrinological, immunological, nutritional, microbial, neuropeptide regulation, in addition to mental health with respect to gut (disease) and vice versa. Neuroanatomically speaking, research is growing increasingly receptive to a possible pathophysiological connection between ASD and IBS. 'Immunogenic' factors such as mastocytosis are showing promising areas for magnetic resonance imaging (MRI) abdominal-pelvic examining, exhibiting increased mental processing (cognitive, visceral motor, and reward-related) interpretation in IBS and ASD.

5. The Gut-Brain Axis: A Key Link

Further, the gut contains the "second brain" or "independent brain," which contains about 500 million neurons (as many as in the spinal cord) because the gut and brain are both originated from the same embryological cells during the fetal life. This gut "independent brain" or "Gut brain," called the enteric nervous system, can perform reflexes without the input from central nervous system because it can work without the CNS in a petri dish. Visceral afferents and humoral signaling within this bidirectional axis are regarded as quite important because the majority (> 90%) of vagal fibers that project from the gut to the brain represent visceral afferents conducting ascending information to the higher centers, such as limbic brain, thalamus, and cortex. After sensory input integration in the CNS, return information may commute to the gut, modifying gastrointestinal motor function, secretion, immune response, or mucosal blood flow. The limbic system and prefrontal cortex are particularly sensitive to this gut-brain interplay and involved symptoms such as vomiting, taste, fullness, bloating, and pain. These pathways serve as a critical interface connecting the emotional and cognitive centers of the brain with peripheral intestinal functions. Modifications in the crosstalk between the brain and gut may affect gut and brain function, contributing to a variety of GI symptoms and sequelae, which translate into clinically identifiable disorders such as functional dyspepsia, restless leg syndrome, autism, and the psychological co-morbidities of the victims of spousal abuse, mental stressors, adaptation of military personnel to wartime activities, and post-traumatic disorder. The relationship between the gut and the brain has been reported to result in the expression of brain-derived neurotropic factor (BDNF) in the mice gut. In addition, pesticides may cross the intestinal barrier and affect the CNS and vice versa.

The gut-brain axis (GBA) is a sophisticated bidirectional system, replete with neural and hormonal signaling pathways that link the gut and brain. The gut-brain crosstalk is managed by the autonomic nervous system (sympathetic and parasympathetic), the neuroendocrine system, and the local immune system. The gut-brain axis represents a relationship between emotional and cognitive centers of the brain with gut functions (gastrointestinal secretions, motility, mucosal permeability, blood flow, and intestinal immunity). The vagal nerve and spinal afferent fibers are essential pathways for communicating information from the gut to the various regions of the brain including the hypothalamus, brainstem, and limbic systems. In addition, the enteric nervous system (gut "brain"), which contains glial cells, endocrine cells producing serotonin, immune cells producing cytokines, as well as neurons, epithelial cells, and connective tissues, is a third division of the autonomic nervous system that participates in the gut-brain axis. Over 90% serotonin and 50% dopamine is present in the gut and 30% gamma aminobutyric acid (GABA) receptors are localized in the enteric nervous system. Thus, many of the same neurochemicals that are found in the central nervous system (CNS) are also present in the enteric nervous system.

5.1. Overview of the Gut-Brain Axis

Due to the fact that there is a complex relationship and constant cross talk among the HPA axis and the gut-brain axis, especially post-puberty, the HPA axis represents a bridge to link many neuropsychiatric disorders to the autistic phenotype. The HPA gland can explain some comorbid psychopathological speculation associated with autism diseases, e.g. SPD, SAD, etc. Whether it is the IBS or the symptoms of autism, both effective or co-effective clinical intervention. Although there is an intricate and integrated regulation of the gut-brain axis, and how the gut, its environment, the functions, and aberrancies are discussed, it is concerned to be the other can contribute to the formation of two central nervous systems, which in turn can culminate in the pathogenesis of IBS-CS and ASD and regression.

As a bi-directional communication network in the human body, the gut-brain axis mediates the central nervous system's regulation of the functions of the gastrointestinal system. By its very nature, the concept of the gut-brain axis illustrates the interconnectedness between the enteric nervous system and the central nervous system. As such, it highlights the fundamental interconnection between the central nervous system and the gastrointestinal system. Of note, Andre Gauriau introduced the concept of brain-gut communication in 1915, and since then, it has been introduced and studied comprehensively in various experimental fields. The impact of gut microbiota in the pathogenesis of Autism Spectrum Disorder (ASD) alongside the contribution of gut-brain interactions in the progression of many neurodevelopmental disorders, including ASD and IBS, has been comprehensively documented. Without a doubt, facing the immunity deformation, disordered energy metabolism, and neurotransmitter imbalance are the different ways various studies highlighted as how ASD and IBS are connected.

5.2. Role in ASD and IBS

Based on the above results, we propose that a main question is to understand the role of the gut in the central disturbance of autism or autism types as found in Down's syndrome. The disturbances in the gut may follow or precede the central disturbances. Irritable bowel syndrome (IBS) in the end is found to form a pharmacological syndrome that does not yet provide possibilities for a good etiology or treatment. Recent studies show that the central disturbances in Down's syndrome (PDD with MD and PDD without MD) may not only include the amygdala, but also connect to both local brain centers (FMR1 and FOXP2). In twins with ASD, a co-variance of gene shared factors was described at the level of symptom severity. Finally, it is clear that the observation in the Jannsen study that paregoric encephalopathy can also include brain growth retardation gives a biological dimension to symptoms describing damage to the gut.

Although the increase in gut permeability and inflammation is typically noted in conditions of IBS, a meta-analysis was able to show that patients with IBS were not more likely to have alimentary comorbidities. This might be due to a milder form of gut permeability and inflammation in IBS that is associated with a disturbed gut barrier function in autism. This normal consequence of autism might improve during intestinal inflammation. Longer studies are necessary to see if the relationship between food intolerance and $\Delta O/N$ (tryptophan) can be used to measure gut inflammation in autism. Prebiotics or probiotics could influence gut inflammation in autism and might improve the combination of IBS with autism. After that, other therapeutic approaches can be analyzed using the gut as a target organ. More research needs to be done to establish the changes that present in the gut and serum either in autism or Down's syndrome.

5.2. Presentation of the role in ASD and IBS

6. Clinical Management and Treatment Approaches

In terms of treatment, it is typically designed at a multisystem approach, which may include working alongside a dietician/nutritionist as well as a psychiatrist/psychologist in some cases. We will discuss a few of the more contemporary approaches.

In our main ASD clinic, we would deliver an abdominal complaint/Bristol chart and only refer it directly to a pediatric gastroenterology team in adults and where the diagnosis of IBS will be in doubt if one or both of the Bristol chart and abdominal complaint has suggested positive findings for IBS. In our secondary clinic for those with a known ASD diagnosis, we offer IBSSS screening unless a history or positive findings are suspected for IBS.

Given the close relationship between Autism Spectrum Disorder (ASD) and Irritable Bowel Syndrome (IBS), we advocate that every patient with ASD, irrespective of symptom status, should undergo investigation for IBS using the Rome IV criteria. This has the potential to minimize distress in autistic individuals and help avoid excessive medical tests to determine the cause of abdominal symptoms, such as upper gastrointestinal endoscopy and colonoscopy, that may present an unacceptable level of great danger and be very distressing when used incorrectly.

Medical interventions for autism, such as alcohol, anticonvulsants, and selective serotonin reuptake inhibitors, have a place in treatment, but there are no approved medications specifically developed for autism. However, antifungal drugs, probiotics, and medications to relax small bowel contractions and manage abdominal pain are commonly prescribed for co-occurring IBS.

Autism and irritable bowel syndrome (IBS) are two complex disorders that are influenced by genetic predispositions and environmental factors. Moreover, they are frequently dismissed as functional disorders, and patients are often told that no treatment is available. This is commonly believed in IBS but is still a common belief in some parts of the autism community. In autism, it can contribute to diagnostic overshadowing, in which clinicians ignore symptoms because they believe they are due to another disorder. In IBS, this may entail a lax approach between the clinician and the patient, which can dissuade the patient from seeking further treatment. It is important and necessary to understand if these concerns need to be undertaken.

6.1. Current Strategies for ASD and IBS

CONCLUSIONS: Based on the present data, there is robust pharmaceutical therapy for treating GI co-morbidities in both ASD and IBS individuals. Effective treatment for active research is less invasive and reverses the GI tract and brain abnormalities in both conditions. Moreover, there is no direct evidence showing current Autism Spectrum Disorder (ASD) therapies in clinical practice contributing to IBS symptoms. RCTs have demonstrated efficacy in pediatric symptoms of IBS (not present in ASD/IBS patients), but aside from few IBS-evening drugs showing behavioral improvements in neurotypical children, have not shown effectiveness on ASD/IBS individuals. However, current strategies might help modulate the abnormal GI signs in ASD/IBS patients several. The current ASD therapies have been centered to other elements of core symptoms, and not to yet fully assessed disparate symptoms such as IBS. Although whether an arrangement for researchers and clinicians to exchange ASD-related IBS ideas or one stop clinic type will be useful still needs to be evaluated.

The connection between Autism Spectrum Disorder (ASD) and Irritable Bowel Syndrome (IBS) is explained in this research article through a comprehensive evaluation. Drawing on the available data, the study demonstrates various treatments and therapies considering Gastrointestinal (GI) symptoms specifically. This can help guide health professionals when presenting management options to the patients and their carers.

6.2. Potential Therapeutic Interventions

Similarly, in ASD, dietary interventions such as casein/gluten-free diets, ketogenic diets, and omega-3 fatty acids have been shown to have positive effects in some cases; however, it is yet to be determined if this is due to improvements in sensory/motor symptoms, GI symptoms, or both. While probiotics and antibiotics are used to treat individuals with ASD and GI symptoms and have shown to be beneficial in IBS patients, further research is needed to determine proper species, dosing, and duration. Microbiome transplants from ASD patients may also be the way of the future. Voluntary hyperventilation is used in IBS patients to increase parasympathetic activity and Bradycardic training Biofeedback as means may in the future improve GI function and symptoms. Gastrointestinal symptoms are commonly seen with the use of selective serotonin reuptake inhibitors (SSRIs), making the connection between disturbed serotonin production in the GI tract and CNS even more apparent than first thought. Treating both autistic symptoms with selective serotonin reuptake inhibitors (SSRIs) and IBS symptoms of anxiety and depression may decrease the severity of their symptoms.

Potential Therapeutic Interventions: Currently, there are no specific medications approved for core symptoms of ASD, but rather symptom-targeting treatments, including aripiprazole and risperidone for irritability and aggression, and the use of Guanfacine for the treatment of hyperactivity, impulsivity, and hyperarousal in ASD.

Typically, therapeutic programs for individuals with ASD will largely consist of behavioral therapies such as Applied Behavior Analysis (ABA), Floortime (DIR Therapy), Son-Rise, and TEACCH. Due to the aforementioned association between GI and autistic-like symptoms, researchers have begun to consider emerging potential treatment approaches used in IBS that may also be useful in IBS comorbid with ASD. A novel approach in IBS therapy examines the use of non-pharmacological dietary interventions, as the gut-brain connection is thought to reside partially in the enteric nervous system using the vagus nerve as a connection.

7. Research Gaps and Future Directions

Two autistic children have a wide comorbidity range, including IBS. However, the pathophysiological connections between the two disorders need further study. As a result, we consider the significance of recognizing the path of the IBD-ASD partnership, given early diagnosis and preventive care, as well as the perceived and likely advantages of the early diagnosis and therapy of IBD in ASD individuals. Identifying and treating the clinical and biological pathways would help minimize the number of IBS cases, thereby reducing the consequences associated with IBS, including the harmful effects of official anti-inflammatory therapy and later immunosuppression. The hospital experience independently documented a much higher prevalence of gastrointestinal comorbidity in people with ASD than in the general population. Understanding the shared biomarkers or genetics across ASD and IBS or IBD, as well as the shared immune- and inflammation-modulating hormones and associated signaling pathways, will be the main headline in addressing future study areas. Future research should comprehensively report the factors that may contribute to the fluctuating severity of gut-brain symptoms as well as gut/gastrointestinal clinical results.

Indeed, there are several challenges when directly comparing results across autism spectrum disorder (ASD) children in different countries, cultures, and communities, all of which introduce variability. As can be seen, the relationship between ASD and irritable bowel syndrome

(IBS) is part of a complex, multifactorial interaction, with immune abnormalities implicated as one potential mediator affecting comorbidities. Research transforming a deeper understanding of the altered connections and abnormalities that arise to associate the ASD population and IBS is necessary and requires unequal interest.

7.1. Challenges in Studying ASD and IBS

Exploring the relationship between ASD and IBS presents two very distinctive features of clinical medicine. First, while defined by the Rome IV criteria, IBS is a diagnosis made purely on the basis of observable phenomena. It is a diagnosis of exclusion and is defined clinically only as the presence of interlinked functional changes in an appropriate biological system (the factors determining which are left unexplained) over a specified time period. Second, the presence of comorbidity with IBS is often described clinically in relation to the depressive sphere of psychiatric disorders, but not in relation to the autism spectrum. As a result, the fact that there is also, potentially, a comorbid relationship between the IBS and ASD, if only via temperamental measures of emotionality, occurs "below the radar".

In stating that Autism Spectrum Disorder (ASD) is "strongly associated with the presence of irritable bowel symptoms," the evidence reviewed in related previous systematic reviews suggests that a comorbid relationship exists. However, while there are small proportions of individuals with ASD who were formally diagnosed with irritable bowel syndrome (IBS), the majority have not had this diagnosis. Moreover, the diagnosis is mediated and limited by the diagnostic and clinical issues identified in the diagnostic rules for this condition. This failure to formally diagnose or understand the condition in ASD also means that we only have a single study on the treatment of IBS in ASD. Thus, as well as justifying further analysis of the comorbid relationship through a method that does not use formal diagnostic boundaries, deep phenotyping, including symptomatology, comorbidity and treatment responses, is ongoing and may increase the possibility of understanding the relationship one day.

7.2. Recommendations for Future Research

In the current article, studies investigating the relationship between IBS and ASD were analysed. The data illustrate a relationship between these two diagnoses, providing new ideas and future goals for studies combining gut and brain pathology. It would be beneficial to carry out studies assessing the relationship between IBS and autism based on paediatric and adult HADS scores.

7.3. Conclusions

The present systematic review has explained research studies for the relationship between ASD and IBS. We have found both preclinical and clinical studies, but to date no experimental study has verified the hypothesis that IBS is correlated with ASD. To the best of our knowledge, there is no experimental study on the therapeutic potential of dietary intervention in ASD children diagnosed with IBS. It is also unknown if dietary interventions could be beneficial for relieving the psychiatric symptoms of ASD. In 2020, Boukthir, Fromentin, Feissy, Saint-Georges, Doppler, Lefevre, Eutamene and Jacquin pointed out that a low-FODMAP diet may help children with ASD and functional abdominal pain. The results were not related to the role of the diet on ASD psychiatric symptoms because their clinical trial sought to evaluate the positive impact of a dietary subgroup. Since 90% of ASD children with functional gastrointestinal disorders also have reported psychiatric symptoms, this small improvement may also contribute to a slight degree in the patient's headache and pain. It is supposed that the search for improved gut and psychiatric symptoms is a link between IBS and ASD. Cognitive behavioural therapy based on gut-directed hypnotherapy achieved better results in reducing bowel symptoms in childhood IBS than in adults, so behavioural therapies may be the first choice for relieving bowel symptoms in ASD children and behavioural discomfort during pain. Possible experimental studies evaluating the reliefs obtained from psychological and dietary interventions on abdominal symptoms experienced by ASD children would reveal how effective psychiatric monitors are on these patients.

7.2. Recommendations for Future Research

8. Conclusion and Implications

Currently, patients with symptoms of either autism or IBS are often referred out of either field of medicine to the favor either GI or neurocognitive complaints. For this reason, if the high comorbidity between autism and IBS in some publications disagrees with the findings of others, it is potential that neuro-cognitive driven GI manifestations may be indistinct in their neural underpinnings from the psychological or somatic driven ones of IBS to provide these clinical statistics. Thus, either associations between these conditions are partially overlapping in terms of the pathways of symptom genesis and for this reason, comorbidities (e.g., asthma) also would need to be investigated at a national level including information on treatments received, age of onset and family history of the symptom.

From the results of the systematic review and critical appraisal, it is clear that the spectrum of ASD is not limited to core social impairments often described in the literature. Substantial functional and visceral comorbidities exist and occur at high rates among individuals with ASD, including features of the GI system. Although existing literature reports the occurrence of IBS and autism at higher rates than expected, the current state of the literature does not provide the tools to accurately measure if an association exists, to describe how this association could emerge, to identify risk factors the two might have in common, or to uncover which core features of either diagnosis are predictive of the other. The classification of autism is under scrutiny, and few advances in the pharmacological treatment of autism have been made. Anti-inflammatory, probiotic, and fecal matter transplant treatments of GI and neurocognitive disorders have generated some promising leads for both disorders. Thus, the symbiotic features of either or both disorders could provide, with future work, some novel pathways that may be therapeutic for both clinical outcomes.

8.1. Summary of Findings

The diagnostic criteria for irritable bowel syndrome (IBS) are lax to nonexistent, since IBS is defined by the caregivers who provide treatment. Not only do the diagnostic criteria lack specificity regarding symptoms, but IBS is also likely not a single condition. Furthermore, multiple comorbidities are seen with IBS. At the same time, there is good justification for proposing that individuals with autism may have significantly related comorbid IBS in which the underlying pathophysiology contributes to soiling and other behaviors often assumed to result from the presence of autism alone. In this project, we studied evidence from the published literature on comorbid ASD and IBS. We found that comorbid IBS in the autism spectrum is common but poorly specified, with little attempt to specify symptom patterns. Both IBS and autism have identified neurological components and produce infections. Thus, we propose an approach to the problem that applies to both nasal and fecal maladies. We also propose studying IBS in ASD.

We have completed a comprehensive analysis of the literature and found a consistent connection between Autism Spectrum Disorder (ASD) and Irritable Bowel Syndrome (IBS) at multiple levels. This connection resides at the level of shared symptoms and symptom clusters, shared etiological risk factors and mechanisms, and shared physiological and molecular mechanisms that produce both conditions and connect them via physiological pathways of acid secretion, inflammation, and gut motility.

We found evidence to support the belief that research on IBS in ASD will benefit individuals on the autism spectrum, but we also found evidence of expanded benefit to the general population. By studying individuals on the autism spectrum without mental impairment, we may gain a unique window into the dynamics of IBS in general. It is our hope that the conclusions we present here will catalyze interested scientists into increased study of IBS in larger samples of people on the autism spectrum with and without intellectual disability.

8.2. Clinical and Research Implications

This research represents the initial comprehensive analysis of the relationship between autism and IBS within a clinical setting and whether any potential co-diagnosis was driven by coexisting GI symptoms. Understanding the high degree of comorbidity between these two conditions may provide a greater understanding of the pathophysiology of autism and IBS. Since autism is assumed to be present prior to any IBS diagnosis, understanding the connection may also have implications for autism causality and treatment options. The relationship between both of these disorders or potentially shared mechanisms relating to GI pain or distress in the brain and gut has been one such line of study. Understanding this will drive autism research and potentially anxiety relieving or neuroinducing therapies. Overall, finding the source of many clinical behaviors and/or aspects of autism that are library controlled is essential and as such understanding may guide research into treatment on potentially controlling autistic behaviors.

This investigation discovered a strong correlation between both autism and irritable bowel syndrome (IBS) and gastrointestinal (GI) symptoms within children with autism. Children with autism had three times the frequency of IBS diagnoses compared to children without autism. This was most often reported between 10 and 20 years of age. This demonstrates the importance of acknowledging the relationship between autism and GI problems and the need for clinical adjustments.

Furthermore, the high correlation creates the possibility of autism being used as an additional diagnostic component for IBS in the future. The single molecule nonpeptide vasoactive intestinal peptide receptor antagonist (NVP018) therapy used to prevent bacterial translocation and brain inflammation in autistic rats may effectively treat autism and IBS.